ALTERNATIVE MEDICINE

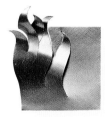

IN A NUTSHELL

ALTERNATIVE MEDICINE
A STEP-BY-STEP GUIDE

ELIZABETH BROWN

ELEMENT

SHAFTESBURY, DORSET • ROCKPORT, MASSACHUSETTS • MELBOURNE, VICTORIA

First published
in Great Britain in 1997 by
ELEMENT BOOKS LIMITED
Shaftesbury,
Dorset, SP7 9BP

Published in the USA in 1997 by
ELEMENT BOOKS INC
PO Box 830, Rockport, MA 01966

Published in Australia in 1997 by
ELEMENT BOOKS LIMITED
and distributed by Penguin Australia Ltd
487 Maroondah Highway, Ringwood,
Victoria 3134

NOTE FROM THE PUBLISHER
Any information given in this book is not
intended to be taken as a replacement for
medical advice. Any person with a
condition requiring medical attention
should consult a qualified practitioner
or therapist.

Designed and created with
The Bridgewater Book Company Ltd

ELEMENT BOOKS LIMITED
Editorial Director Julia McCutchen
Managing Editor Caro Ness
Project Editor Allie West
Production Director Roger Lane
Production Sarah Golden

THE BRIDGEWATER BOOK COMPANY
Art Director Kevin Knight
Designers Andrew Milne, Jane Lanaway
Managing Editor Anne Townley
Project Co-ordinator Fiona Corbridge
Page layout Chris Lanaway
Picture Research Lynda Marshall
Three-dimensional models Mark Jamieson
Photography Ian Parsons, Guy Ryecart
Illustrations Andrew Milne, Pip Adams

Text consultants BOOK CREATION SERVICES LTD
Series Editor Karen Sullivan

Printed and bound by Dai Nippon, Hong Kong

British Library Cataloguing in
Publication data available

Library of Congress Cataloging
in Publication data available

ISBN 1-86204-155-5

The publishers wish to thank the
following for the use of pictures:
Bridgeman Art Library, e.t. archive,
Mansell Collection, The Society of Teachers
of the Alexander Technique, and Zefa.

Special thanks go to:
Jean Begley, Paul Castle, Natasha
Gray, Jo Mortimer
for help with photography.

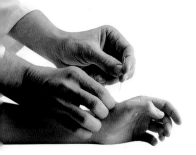

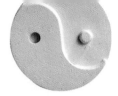

Contents

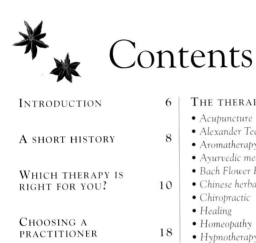

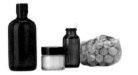

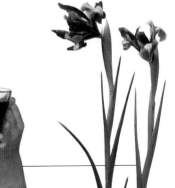

Introduction

OVER THE PAST *few decades, we have become overly dependent upon modern medicine for all our health needs. We have grown used to the comfort of having a physician prescribe medication for every symptom of ill-health, and we no longer question the cause of those symptoms. There is, today, virtually a pill for all ills, and we have grown to expect just that.*

ABOVE **Our choice:** *alternative or conventional medicine.*

Modern medicine is indeed marvelous in many ways, and many of us would not be alive without it. But some problems can be prevented if we take more responsibility for our own health. That means recognizing the symptoms of ill-health, and treating minor complaints before they become full-blown illnesses.

RIGHT
The holistic approach to good health gives equal consideration to different aspects of lifestyle.

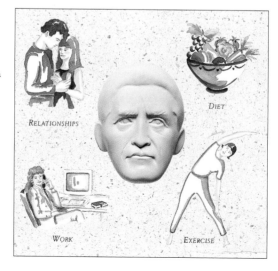

RELATIONSHIPS

DIET

WORK

EXERCISE

Our doctors and health services are overstretched, and there is little time to analyze a patient's problems. The symptoms are resolved with whatever medication best fits the bill, and most patients are in and out of their physicians' offices within five minutes. Studies show that more than 70 per cent of those patients come out with a prescription. Obviously five minutes is not enough time to understand that, perhaps, the real cause of someone's headaches is an inability to sleep caused by the death of a loved one a year earlier.

This is where holistic medicine comes in – the foundation of most alternative therapies. Alternative therapists believe that we are the sum of all our parts – that it is our emotions, lifestyles, and overall constitutions which are the root causes of ill-health. Alternative practitioners have time to explore these factors instead of just treating symptoms and the complaint alone.

Alternative therapies should not be considered a replacement for conventional medicine, but the two should work hand in hand.

These various therapies are vastly different, and each calls upon the medical practices of other cultures, which may treat illness and health in a completely different way.

Holistic medicine addresses not only the whole person, but also the person's environment, and involves various healing and health-promoting practices. Holistic practitioners believe that patients should be active participants in their own health care, since all individuals are seen to have the capacity – mental, emotional, social, spiritual, and physical – to heal themselves.

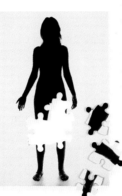

ABOVE *Like a jigsaw, good health consists of interlocking elements.*

A short history

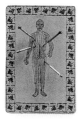

ABOVE **The meridian lines feature in Chinese medicine**

MOST OF OUR *knowledge comes from the writings of the ancient Indians, Chinese, Greeks, Romans, and Egyptians, who were both practitioners and avid documenters of the medical discoveries of their age. As armies and travelers moved around the world, their medical skills, their plants, and other forms of medicine went with them. These complemented the various practices of healing they encountered on their travels and led to the development and refinement of their treatments. Today we have a vast array of therapies to choose from, originating from all over the world (look at the map on the right).*

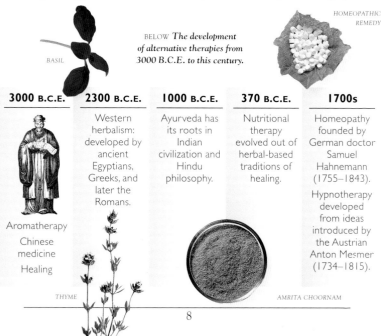

HOMEOPATHIC REMEDY

BELOW **The development of alternative therapies from 3000 B.C.E. to this century.**

BASIL

3000 B.C.E.	2300 B.C.E.	1000 B.C.E.	370 B.C.E.	1700s
	Western herbalism: developed by ancient Egyptians, Greeks, and later the Romans.	Ayurveda has its roots in Indian civilization and Hindu philosophy.	Nutritional therapy evolved out of herbal-based traditions of healing.	Homeopathy founded by German doctor Samuel Hahnemann (1755–1843).
Aromatherapy Chinese medicine Healing				Hypnotherapy developed from ideas introduced by the Austrian Anton Mesmer (1734–1815).

THYME

AMRITA CHOORNAM

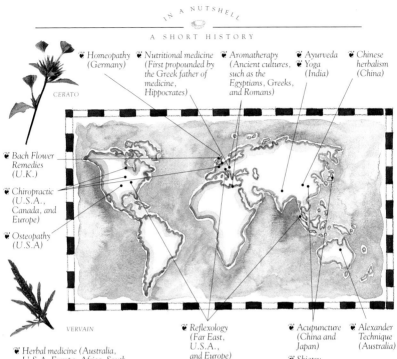

Homeopathy (Germany)

Nutritional medicine (First propounded by the Greek father of medicine, Hippocrates)

Aromatherapy (Ancient cultures, such as the Egyptians, Greeks, and Romans)

Ayurveda Yoga (India)

Chinese herbalism (China)

CERATO

Bach Flower Remedies (U.K.)

Chiropractic (U.S.A., Canada, and Europe)

Osteopathy (U.S.A)

VERVAIN

Herbal medicine (Australia, U.S.A, Europe, Africa, South America, India, China, Japan)

Reflexology (Far East, U.S.A., and Europe)

Acupuncture (China and Japan)

Shiatsu (Japan)

Alexander Technique (Australia)

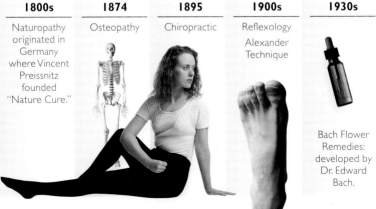

1800s	1874	1895	1900s	1930s
Naturopathy originated in Germany where Vincent Preissnitz founded "Nature Cure."	Osteopathy	Chiropractic	Reflexology Alexander Technique	Bach Flower Remedies: developed by Dr. Edward Bach.

9

Which therapy is right for you?

JASMINE

THE VARIETY of therapies available presents a bewildering choice. Many therapies, such as Ayurveda, homeopathy, acupuncture, and reflexology, are systems of medicine that include diet, lifestyle, and medical attention. For a beginner, or someone with a chronic, long-standing health problem, these might prove to be the most useful, outlining exactly how to change your lifestyle in order to achieve optimum health and well-being.

CASE STUDY

❋ John was troubled by catarrh after a succession of colds during the winter.

❋ A homeopath prescribed Ant. tart. remedy. She also recommended that John gave himself more time to relax.

❋ A nutritional therapist advised a complete re-think of John's diet, which consisted of a lot of fast foods. He prescribed a vitamin and mineral supplement.

If you cringe at the thought of needles, acupuncture may not be for you – but acupressure, which involves working the same points with pressure rather than needles, may be more suitable. The therapies section (pages 22 to 53) outlines what is available, along with the basic theories and details of what each therapy can treat. Look through to see what appeals to you.

Many therapies can be combined – aromatherapy is complementary to most other therapies, except homeopathy, which may be

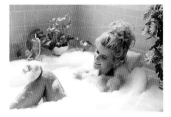

ABOVE *Aromatherapy oils added to bubble bath will not conflict with other treatments.*

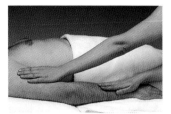

ABOVE *Massage is beneficial for many aches and pains.*

affected by some of the more powerful oils. As a rule of thumb, try one therapy at a time so you know which one works. Add others when you have found one that you like. You may find that Chinese herbalism controls your eczema, but you like to have your spirits lifted by the occasional osteopathic treatment or aromatherapy bath. That's perfectly acceptable. The whole point of alternative therapies is that you are taking charge of your own health, and by ensuring that your sense of well-being is the best it can be, you will attain good health on every level.

RIGHT *Yoga combines physical and spiritual aspects for good health.*

WHAT TO EXPECT FROM ALTERNATIVE THERAPIES

You will be expected to give a complete picture of your health and lifestyle in order for your therapist to make an informed decision about the course of your treatment. The cause of your symptoms will be investigated and dealt with, not just the symptoms themselves. You can expect your symptoms to become worse, occasionally, before they get better, which is a sign that your body is responding to treatment and beginning to help itself. The basis of all alternative therapies is that they stimulate your body to heal itself.

WHAT CONDITIONS CAN BE TREATED?

Almost all conditions can be treated by alternative medicine, some more successfully than others. Stress and related conditions are usually dealt with very efficiently because most systems strive to ensure that your health is at optimum level, that your immune system is strong, and that you are feeling relaxed. With a strong immune system, you will find you become ill less often, and that when you do come down with something, you fight it off much more quickly and efficiently.

Medical emergencies must always be addressed by a qualified physician. Alternative medicine is not a replacement for conventional medicine, but a complement to it. Make sure you tell your physician about any alternative treatments you are receiving, and tell your alternative health practitioner about any conventional medication that you are taking.

Sarah Smith
1512 Johnson Drive

Physician : Dr Anthony Green
No major illnesses or operations
Not on any medication

Reasons for consultation
Inability to lose weight
Problems sleeping

A THERAPIST'S
PATIENT RECORD

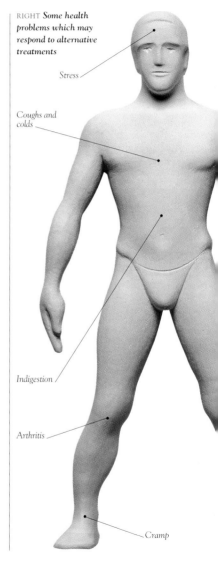

RIGHT *Some health problems which may respond to alternative treatments*

Stress

Coughs and colds

Indigestion

Arthritis

Cramp

DO ALTERNATIVE THERAPIES WORK?

There is a great deal of contemporary research into the efficacy of alternative therapies. There is no question that most of them do work, although modern science has had difficulty in justifying that on a scientific level. Spiritual healing, for instance, works for thousands and thousands of people each year, and in some cases terminal illnesses have been cured. There is no explanation for how this has happened, but we do know that it has.

Some therapies require more of a leap of faith – for instance Bach Flower Remedies, or homeopathy. Others are similar to conventional Western medicine, in that you take medication for a complaint. Some people believe that alternative therapies work because the patient is able to spend so much time in consultation with the practitioner, which is in itself therapeutic. But this doesn't explain the fact that most of the therapies listed in this book work on infants, babies, and people who are no longer able to think for themselves. Some therapies will work for you, some may not. Experiment and enjoy the whole process!

ROSE PETALS

Varicose veins

LEFT *Your therapist will take a detailed case history at your first consultation.*

OUR BODIES

Our bodies comprise the systems listed below, all of which work together to undertake body processes.

BODY SYSTEMS

- Circulatory system.
- Respiratory system.
- Mind, brain, and nervous system.
- Endocrine system.
- Reproductive system (male).
- Reproductive system (female).
- Urinary system (male and female).
- Digestive system.
- Immune (lymphatic) system.
- Eyes.
- Ears, nose, throat, and mouth.
- Skin (and hair).
- Musculoskeletal system.

Alternative therapies focus on balancing these systems so that they work efficiently. Much attention is given to the immune system, which is responsible for fighting infection. An efficient immune system is crucial to good health, and most

complementary therapy treatment is aimed at improving or boosting a system that may be flagging, or is impaired by any one of a number of problems. The premise that prevention is always better than cure is fundamental to complementary medicine, and the immune system is the ideal place to begin preventative treatment. A healthy immune system

ABOVE **The circulatory system: the heart pumps blood around the body.**

ABOVE **The endocrine system releases hormones into the bloodstream.**

prevents you from being hampered by illness, will allow you to fight off infections and allergies, and will ensure that you recover from illness quickly and readily.

Most of the therapies listed in this book will boost your immune system and will ensure the smooth running of other body systems.

ENEMIES

Your immune system can be impaired by the following factors:

- Injuries.
- Surgery.
- The overuse of antibiotics.
- Some drugs.
- Digestive disorders.
- Poor diet.
- Pollution.
- Stress.
- Genetic problems.
- Disease.
- Inherited weaknesses.

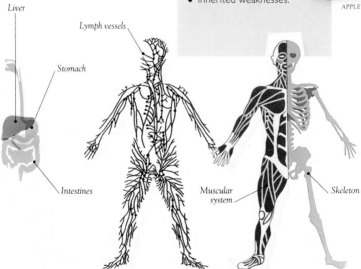

APPLE

Liver

Lymph vessels

Stomach

Intestines

Muscular system

Skeleton

ABOVE **The digestive system: food is broken down and absorbed.**

ABOVE **The lymphatic system carries excess fluid and other particles.**

ABOVE **The musculoskeletal system: our basic framework.**

USING ALTERNATIVE THERAPIES ALONGSIDE ORTHODOX TREATMENT

Most therapies can be undertaken alongside conventional medical treatment, but you must advise your physician of any treatment you are receiving elsewhere. Some conventional drugs will nullify alternative treatments, such as certain homeopathic remedies. Some conditions may be affected by herbs or oils. Your physician may know a little about alternative therapies, and may perhaps even use some. Ask for a referral to an alternative practitioner. Homeopathy, chiropractic, nutritional medicine, and osteopathy are now considered mainstream and generally approved by much of the conventional medical establishment.

If you suffer from a chronic illness or are pregnant, consult a physician before beginning any alternative treatment.

REMEMBER

Your alternative practitioner will need to know if you are taking any medication.

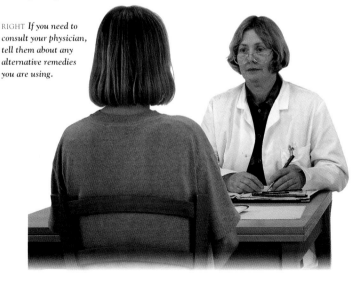

RIGHT *If you need to consult your physician, tell them about any alternative remedies you are using.*

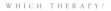
SAFETY NOTES

ROSEMARY

Some therapies are not suitable for certain age groups and health conditions, and you must tell your therapist if you suffer from any medical complaints. Some aromatherapy oils can bring on contractions in a pregnant woman, which could cause miscarriage. Certain bone diseases must never be treated with osteopathy or chiropractic, and your practitioner must be aware of any health conditions in order to suggest the best possible treatment. Babies, children, and the elderly will all respond to the majority of therapies, depending on the severity of their condition, although some therapies are more suitable than others. Conditions such as colic and hyperactivity in children, menopausal complaints, and degenerative diseases have no conventional cures, but have been successfully treated with alternative therapies.

Alternative medicine improves your sense of well-being, so that even if a long-standing problem takes some time to cure, you will feel so much better generally, that other annoying complaints disappear as well.

> CAUTION
>
> Always consult a trained, qualified, and registered practitioner and ask to see evidence of qualifications.

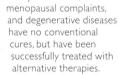

LEFT **If you plan to experiment with different therapies, tell each practitioner about the treatments you are undertaking.**

A good therapist will ask you about all aspects of your lifestyle and feelings. He or she will thoroughly examine every aspect of your health and listen carefully to what you say.

REGISTERED QUALIFIED PRACTITIONER

LEFT **Thyme oil should not be used in pregnancy.**

ABOVE **Look for a qualified therapist.**

Choosing a practitioner

THE SUCCESS *of alternative therapies can be enormously dependent on a good practitioner/ patient relationship, and your choice of a therapist is as important as the choice of therapy. Take your time, check the therapist's qualifications, ask for recommendations from friends, your physician, or another therapist, and do not commit yourself until you are sure you will have a rapport. Because you will be imparting a great deal of information about yourself, you must feel that you can be honest.*

The following steps will help you in your choice:
- Choose your therapy.
- Ring the organization or association of the therapy in which you are interested for a list of practitioners, or ask your physician or other therapist for a recommendation.
- Speak to your practitioner on the telephone, and if you are happy, make an appointment.
- Find out about qualifications and experience.

- Establish whether or not you feel you will be able to get along with the therapist. Instinct is of prime importance here.
- The therapist should be supportive and helpful, but not intrusive.
- Remember that prices vary enormously between one therapist and another. Some therapies are very expensive. Always find out what you will get for your money.

THE CONSULTATION

The consultation is the most important part of any alternative therapy session. This is the first session with a therapist, and the one in which the most information is exchanged. The first session usually lasts longer than any subsequent sessions because your therapist will aim to find out all about you, as well as your problem, before any diagnosis can be made. You can expect your therapist to question you on the areas below. With this information, your therapist can go ahead and make a diagnosis, which forms the next part of the consultation.

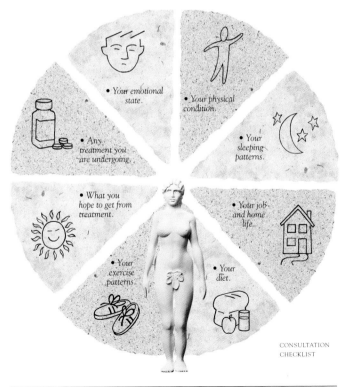

- Your emotional state.
- Your physical condition.
- Any treatment you are undergoing.
- Your sleeping patterns.
- What you hope to get from treatment.
- Your job and home life.
- Your exercise patterns.
- Your diet.

CONSULTATION CHECKLIST

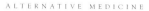
Diagnostic techniques

EVERY DISCIPLINE *has different techniques for finalizing a diagnosis. In Chinese medicine, for instance, your practitioner will look at your tongue, take a number of pulses, palpate your body, and assess you just by looking at different parts of your body. With that information, he or she will prescribe for you a course of treatment.*

ABOVE **The tongue is an indicator of health.**

Some diagnostic techniques include:
• Iridology (viewing the eyes as a map of the body and pinpointing any weaknesses in the irises).
• Kinesiology (muscle tests that display body health).

• Kirlian photography (photographing the quality of the energy of a person, which is altered where there is imbalance).
• Biofeedback (monitoring responses to various physical tests by machine).

COMPARING DIAGNOSTIC TECHNIQUES

Many physical therapies will be able to locate problem areas in the process of an examination – a reflexologist will, for instance, be able to tell a lot about your physical condition by your response to her finger pressure on your feet. A sensitivity indicates an imbalance in the related systems (see page 48). An iridologist also uses a map of

the eyes, correlating flecks on the iris with problems in the body. Other, less physical systems, such as homeopathy, may diagnose on the basis of your verbal communication.

HOW TO JUDGE THE RESULTS

Many people do not seek out alternative therapies until they have become thoroughly disillusioned by the conventional medical system, and by then, many long-standing conditions have become quite deeply entrenched. It is normal for treatments to take some time. They are not miracle cures, but gentle and effective means of encouraging your body to work for itself.

Many therapies initiate a process of detoxification, when you may suffer from headaches, dizziness, poor skin, rashes, diarrhea, nausea, and discharge. This is normal and you may find that symptoms become worse or change as your treatment progresses. This shows that your body is hard at work.

If you experience no change in your condition, you should go back to your therapist. Always give your therapist a second chance: diagnosis is extremely complicated and you may have

LEFT *Iridology and reflexology relate areas of the eyes and feet respectively to parts of the body.*

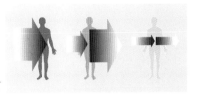

ABOVE *After detoxification, the body expels as many toxins as it takes in.*

unknowingly omitted a major piece of information that changes the whole treatment picture. If several attempts to effect a cure fail completely, you may think about trying a different therapy, or therapist.

COMPLAINTS PROCEDURES

All therapies have governing bodies and associations that usually try to ensure the reputation of their discipline. They will have names of registered, qualified therapists, and if you do have a complaint, take it straight to the regulatory board. Some therapies do not require professional qualifications, but all good therapists should be able to show evidence of their training, and should belong to a recognized board. If your therapist does not belong to one, send your complaint to their training college or faculty. If you are genuinely unhappy with treatment, your money should be refunded.

Acupuncture

ACUPUNCTURE IS *a traditional Chinese medical treatment, in which a number of very fine metal needles are inserted into the skin at any of the 800 specially designated points. The word "acupuncture" means "needle piercing," and involves the use of many elements of traditional Chinese medicine, including Chinese herbalism, massage, moxabustion (see right), and diet and lifestyle changes. In China it has long been used for pain relief and treatment of such ailments as arthritis, high blood-pressure, and ulcers.*

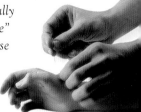

ABOVE **A point farthest from the site of the symptoms is needled, as well as local points.**

Acupuncture is said to work by manipulating the body's energy flow, called "chi," allowing the body to balance and heal itself. Chi travels through meridians in the body, and where it becomes blocked or stagnant, disease or ill-health can exist. An acupuncturist will pinpoint a weakness in your chain of energy, or chi, and treat it according to your symptoms or "pattern of disharmony."

Chi is the unique force that enables our bodies to function on every level. It flows through invisible meridians, each of which is named after and related to an organ, including the lung, kidney, stomach, spleen, and heart.

Relieves indigestion, weak bladder, backache.

LEFT **Needling the stomach and bladder channels to build up chi.**

Meridians run through many parts of the body, and every point along a specific meridian will be affected by any disharmony at other points. For example, the teeth are part of the stomach meridian. Teething babies may therefore also suffer digestive disorders.

You should feel a tingling sensation when the needle penetrates the skin: if you feel nothing, it is unlikely that the correct acupuncture point has been needled.

Two other related techniques are moxabustion and cupping.

• Moxabustion involves burning herbs, or "moxa," at specific acupuncture points. It is used to warm and stimulate chi.

• Cupping involves the use of a warmed cup, which is placed upside-down on a specific acupuncture point. It creates a vacuum to draw the blood and energy to that point.

RIGHT **Moxabustion stimulates energy in areas of weak chi.**

IS IT SAFE?

Acupuncture is safe for people of every age and of all levels of health. Ensure that your practitioner is qualified, and that disposable needles are used.

TREATMENT

❄ **Problems treated**
Stress, depression, pain, addictions, childbirth, M.E., allergies, asthma and eczema, injuries, fatigue, digestive disorders, circulatory disorders, menstrual problems, sexual problems, infertility.

❄ **Number of sessions necessary**
Once or twice a week to begin with, then weekly until the condition clears. It is often suggested that you return every one or two months to rebalance your system as a preventive measure.

ACUPRESSURE

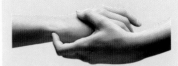

Acupressure involves the use of finger pressure on acupuncture points, to stimulate the smooth flow of chi through the energy channels of the body. It involves mostly thumb and fingertip pressure, although it can also incorporate massage along the meridians.

Alexander Technique

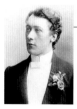

ABOVE *Frederick Alexander.*

THE ALEXANDER TECHNIQUE, *created by Frederick Alexander, an Australian actor, focuses on the fundamental belief that by correcting the way the body is held and used, physical and psychological well-being can be enhanced. Alexander believed that by becoming more aware of our bodies – our posture, balance, and movement in everyday activities – bad habits which had developed over time could be discarded. In this way, natural motion would be restored, along with proper functioning of the body.*

Alexander retaught posture and basic control of the body. The technique enables students to differentiate between uncontrolled, unnecessary effort, and natural freedom of movement – which allows the body to function at optimum level. Incorrect posture and misuse of the body cause it to sag, which leads to the distortion of the spinal curves, and causes muscles to shorten and become stiff. The resulting tendencies are strain, headaches, stiffness, fatigue, backaches, and a general malaise.

The Alexander Technique is not a therapy as such, but a process of re-education which allows us to rediscover our natural poise, grace and freedom, and use our bodies more efficiently. It is often referred to as "posture training," and it is taught in lessons where the practitioner is referred to as a teacher.

ABOVE *Always be aware of your posture and try to eliminate bad habits.*

The Alexander Technique focuses on training you to work out the distortions in your body, and encourage natural reflexes to work once again. Muscle tone is improved and the body becomes relaxed enough to release tension, improve breathing, circulation, and digestion. Posture and balance are improved, making breathing easier. Movement becomes more natural and poised, and harmful pressures on organs and body systems are released.

Overall, the Alexander Technique is aimed at encouraging awareness of the body, so that you have an increased sense of confidence, greater vitality, and an improved, positive mental outlook. Improved physical health will also result.

IS IT SAFE?

The technique is safe for people of all ages, and indeed many elderly people and pregnant women benefit from treatment. The body can be re-educated to correct posture and generally improve health.

TREATMENT

❋ Problems treated
Sessions are aimed at improving overall posture and body responses, and many conditions respond to this, particularly those such as asthma, headaches, eczema, and fatigue, which are exacerbated by stress. Circulatory problems, breathing disorders, and musculoskeletal conditions may respond to treatment, although the Alexander Technique does not set out to "cure" as such, rather to encourage body systems to work more effectively.

❋ Number of sessions necessary
The Alexander Technique is quite complex, and usually 25 to 45 lessons are required to learn the processes involved. The sessions are, however, very therapeutic, and many people carry on indefinitely.

LEFT *The correct way to sit on a chair (right), with straight back and feet flat on the floor.*

Aromatherapy

AROMATHERAPY *is a combination of two words: "aroma," which means smell or fragrance; and "therapy," which means a treatment for the body, mind, or social condition of a person, to assist or facilitate a process where healing and change can take place.*

ESSENTIAL OIL

Aromatherapy uses essential oils, which are the "life force" of aromatic flowers, herbs, plants, trees, or spices. Each oil has individual qualities which work toward restoring balance within the body.

When the oils come into contact with the skin, they may stimulate nerve endings, circulation, the lymphatic system, muscles, tissues, the nervous system, or endocrine activity.

When oils are inhaled, they stimulate nerve endings in the nose, and messages are carried to the brain.

RIGHT **Aromatherapy uses gentle forms of massage.**

IS IT SAFE?

Many oils are contraindicated by medical conditions: consult a physician if you suffer from a long-term health problem, are pregnant, or are taking medication. Some oils are unsuitable for babies.

TREATMENT

❋ **Problems treated**
Aromatherapy is "holistic," meaning it is aimed at balancing the whole person — mind, body, and spirit. For this reason, almost any health condition can be improved by aromatherapy. It is extremely effective for stress and its related disorders, muscular problems, emotional disorders, female complaints such as menopause, pregnancy, and period problems, digestive disorders, and skin problems.

❋ **Number of sessions necessary**
Many conditions will respond immediately, but depending on the severity of the problem, and the length of time you have had it, up to 10 sessions may be necessary.

DOG ROSE

ROSEMARY

COMMONLY USED OILS

Lavender Relaxing, healing, analgesic, antidepressant, deodorant, diuretic, insecticidal, nervine, tonic, sedative, stimulant. Lavender is adaptogenic: uplifting if you are tired, and relaxing if you are stressed.

Thyme Antioxidant, antiseptic, antispasmodic, astringent, diuretic, expectorant, stimulant, tonic.

Eucalyptus Antiseptic, antiviral, bactericidal, deodorant, expectorant, fungicidal, insecticidal.

Chamomile Analgesic, anti-allergenic, anti-inflammatory, antispasmodic, bactericidal, digestive, brings down fever, nervine, sedative, relaxing.

Rose Antidepressant, antiseptic, antispasmodic, bactericidal, sedative, tonic (heart, liver, stomach, and uterus), laxative, hepatic.

Rosemary Warming, stimulating, analgesic, antiseptic, nervine, tonic, antispasmodic, diuretic, hypertensive.

LAVENDER FLOWERS

USING ESSENTIAL OILS

Massage: with oils diluted in a suitable carrier oil.

Bath: a few drops in the bath will work by inhalation and will allow the oils to be absorbed through the skin.

Steam inhalation: put a few drops of essential oil in hot water and inhale.

Vaporizer: place oil in a burner or on a light bulb to allow the heat to release the essential qualities into the air.

Compress: essential oil can be applied to an affected area on a cotton compress – warm or cold.

Cream, lotion, shampoo, shower gel: essential oils can be added for extra benefit.

Gargle, mouthwash: some oils are suitable for internal use, and can be used in a gargle or rinse.

Using neat: some essential oils can be applied undiluted to the skin.

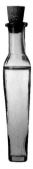

ABOVE
Eucalyptus oil is good for inhalation.

Ayurvedic medicine

AYURVEDIC MEDICINE *is the traditional, all-embracing national system of medicine practiced in India and Sri Lanka. Like traditional Chinese medicine, Ayurveda is a comprehensive system of healthcare with many elements working together to provide guidance for living. It is a way of life aimed at good health, rather than a treatment for specific illnesses.*

ABOVE **Ayurveda aims to obviate the need for orthodox medicine.**

WATER

FIRE

The basic Ayurvedic belief is that everything within the universe, including ourselves, is composed of energy or "prana." By balancing that energy within ourselves and in relation to the world around us, we will promote health on all levels.

Ayurvedic practitioners believe that we are composed of constantly changing energy. Ayurveda teaches us how to encourage the balance of energy, which controls the functions of every cell in our bodies. That means our thoughts, feelings, actions, food, sleeping patterns, relationships,

RIGHT **Yoga addresses both physical and spiritual health.**

RIGHT **Energy has five elements: earth, air, fire, water, and space.**

ELEMENTS

Some of the elements of Ayurvedic medicine include:

- A type of aromatherapy.
- Breathing.
- Detoxification.
- Diet.
- Exercise.
- Herbs.
- Manipulation of vital energy points (called marma).
- Meditation.
- Music therapy.
- Techniques aimed at emotional and psychological health.
- Yoga.

ABOVE **Herbs such as jethimade are used in Ayurvedic medicine.**

personal habits, and fears – and everything else that is a part of us – affect our energy levels, the quality of that energy, and through that our health itself.

Ayurvedic practitioners often work on the immune system, in order to balance energies and keep it strong so that it is able to fight invaders and relieve chronic conditions. There are several main constitutional types, and once yours is established, you are given a set of guidelines to follow, which are an individually prepared plan for health, mind, and spiritual maintenance.

Ayurvedic principles are based on the belief that we are composed of combinations of five elements: air, fire, space, water, and earth. There are then three other forces called vata, pitta, and kapha in which the five elements are manifest. Health can only be achieved when all the forces are balanced.

IS IT SAFE?

Ayurveda is safe for people of all levels of health. Some of the treatments will be altered for people with health conditions, pregnant women, and children. Certain conditions such as cancer, some hernias, and mechanical problems, are not suitable for Ayurvedic treatments.

TREATMENT

❋ Problems treated

Ayurvedic medicine can, in theory, address any type of health problem, and is particularly useful for shifting long-term or chronic conditions. In particular, allergies, digestive disorders, anxiety, depression, headaches, insomnia, respiratory problems, skin problems, stress, and high blood-pressure respond.

❋ Number of sessions necessary

Most conditions will respond in between three and ten visits, depending on their severity and how long they have been a problem.

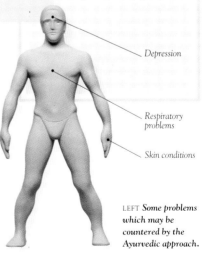

Depression

Respiratory problems

Skin conditions

LEFT *Some problems which may be countered by the Ayurvedic approach.*

Bach Flower Remedies

BACH FLOWER REMEDIES *use the life essence of flowers to balance the negative emotions that lead to, and are symptoms of, disease. They are a natural method of establishing personal equilibrium and harmony. Edward Bach, a Welsh homeopath and bacteriologist, formulated the remedies, which are simple to make and use and can be safely taken by people of all ages and conditions.*

Bach believed there was a crucial relationship between the mental outlook of a person and their physical state. He stated that negative emotions could manifest themselves physically as pain, stress, and also as illness.

Bach Flower Remedies heal the mind in a gentle, natural

The 38 Bach Flower Remedies

Agrimony For those who hide their feelings.

Aspen For fear of the unknown.

Beech For the perfectionist who finds it hard to tolerate the shortcomings of others.

Centaury For those who are kind, gentle and eager to please, and who find it impossible to say no.

Cerato For those who seek the reassurance of others because they do not trust their own judgment or intuition.

Cherry Plum For those who feel anxious, and overwhelmingly depressed.

Chestnut bud For those who keep making the same mistakes, never seeming to learn from past experiences.

Chicory For the mothering type who is loving, but overprotective and possessive.

Clematis For the artistic dreamer, who may lack concentration.

Crabapple For those who feel infected or unclean, revolted by eating, or sex, or who have a hygiene fixation.

Elm For those who are overwhelmed by pressure from work, family, and other commitments.

Gentian For those who are easily discouraged. Even when they are doing well, small setbacks dishearten them.

Gorse For those who believe that they were born to suffer and are pessimistic about everything.

Heather For those who always talk about themselves, so nobody else can get a word in.

Holly For those who are overcome with suspicion. Also for hatred, jealousy, and the desire for revenge.

Honeysuckle For those who dwell on the past to the extent that they lose interest in the present.

Hornbeam For those who are mentally exhausted at the thought of work.

Impatiens For those who do everything in a hurry. They are brusque, finish sentences for people, fidget, and edge toward the door when others are still talking.

---

way, ensuring that the body has the will to heal itself and to right any imbalances.

There are 38 Bach Flower Remedies developed to support every conceivable personality, attitude, and negative state of mind. They were developed as a complete system and, before his death, Bach gave instructions that no more remedies were to be added to the set.

LARCH

TREATMENT

❈ **Problems treated**
Any emotional or mental condition. In particular, stress, digestive disorders, sleep problems, and skin problems tend to respond well.

❈ **Number of sessions necessary**
One or two sessions is usually enough to diagnose negative qualities and treat them accordingly. Some conditions may require more sessions.

IS IT SAFE?

Bach Flower Remedies are safe for people of every age and state of health, and will not interfere with any other medication.

VERVAIN

Larch For those with ability but no confidence, missing opportunities because of self-doubt and feelings of inferiority.

Mimulus For those who are shy, nervous, and blush easily.

Mustard For those who are gloomy for no apparent reason.

Oak For the fighter who never gives in.

Olive For those who are exhausted due to overwork or over-exertion.

Pine For those who feel guilty, even when it is not their fault.

Red Chestnut For those who are over-anxious for family and friends, and are afraid of impending disaster.

Rock Rose For terror or panic, which may not be rational.

Rock Water For those who are strict with themselves, and demand perfection.

Scleranthus For emotional distress due to indecision.

Star of Bethlehem For the inconsolable after shock, bereavement, or bad news.

Sweet Chestnut For those in utter despair.

Vervain For the enthusiastic, talkative, principled perfectionist who is incensed by injustice and fights for the underdog.

Vine For the leader: strong, dominant, ambitious, and determined, but sometimes tyrannical.

Walnut For change. It settles people into a new environment, and helps cope with life changes.

Water Violet For the reserved, self-contained, and dignified, who may be aloof.

White Chestnut For those who are tormented by persistent worries and unwanted thoughts.

Wild Oat For those who are dithering at a crossroads in life.

Wild Rose For those who drift and have no enthusiasm to change any aspect of their life.

Willow For the grouchy, introspective pessimist, who wallows in self-pity.

Rescue Remedy The most frequently used of all the remedies is Rescue Remedy, a "composite" remedy, made up of Star of Bethlehem, Rock Rose, Impatiens, Cherry Plum, and Clematis.

Chinese herbalism

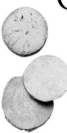

CHINESE HERBALISM *is the use of herbs to treat and prevent physical and emotional ill-health. The Chinese herbal tradition dates back more than 3,000 years, and ancient pharmacopeia detailing herbs and their effects still exist today. The herbs may be in raw form or processed into pills, powders, ointments, liquid tonics, or teas. They are classified according to their properties. The majority are of plant origin but a few are from mineral sources or from animal products.*

ABOVE *Ze xie, or water plantain tuber.*

XIN YI HUA

Traditional Chinese diagnostic techniques are used to determine the cause of ill-health and "patterns of disharmony" in the body. Herbs are prescribed to restore harmony to mind, body, and emotions. They mainly improve immunity and support, and balance the healing system, rather than kill disease. However, certain herbs can also be prescribed to fight infection.

The Chinese believe that each one of us is governed by the opposing, but complementary, forces of yin and yang. They also believe that "chi" is the energy that binds yin and yang. When chi is unbalanced, it can lead to illness. Chi flows through channels called meridians. Herbalism allows chi to flow smoothly, restoring harmony to the whole person.

Through a detailed system of diagnosis, the Chinese herbalist can identify the

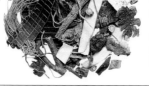

LEFT *There are over 10,000 ways in which herbs can be combined.*

YIN YANG SYMBOL

root cause of imbalance. Herbs are prescribed specifically for the meridian responsible for the imbalance, to rebalance chi and the associated element. The effect that a particular herb exerts on the meridian depends on its properties.

Herbs have different properties, which means they can restore warmth to cold chi, move stagnant chi, or slow chi. Herbs are usually defined according to their properties and how they work in the body.

Herbs also have their own particular tastes, each of which affects a different organ and element. The herbs are never prescribed alone, but in combinations of up to 12 at a time. They combine to complement, assist, moderate, and modify the actions of each other, and in some cases to counteract each other's side-effects so that the patient suffers no ill-effects from a particularly strong herb.

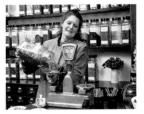

ABOVE **Weighing out herbs at a specialist herb supplier.**

TREATMENT

❀ Problems treated
Chinese herbs can be used for a wide range of ailments including asthma, skin diseases, menstrual problems, neurological disorders, infertility, allergies, arthritis, depression, digestive disturbances, and migraine. They are effective when used on their own or in conjunction with another therapy such as acupuncture.

SHI CHANG PU

❀ Number of sessions necessary
Chronic illness may take several weeks of regular treatment for healing to take place; acute ailments may respond immediately.

IS IT SAFE?

If prescribed by qualified and experienced practitioners and used properly, these herbs rarely cause side-effects and can provide very effective treatment.

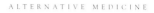

Chiropractic

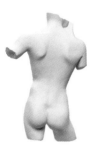

CHIROPRACTIC IS A *medical practice based on the theory that disease results from a disruption of nerve function. This interference is thought to stem primarily from displaced vertebrae, which chiropractors massage and manipulate manually in order to relieve pressure on nerves.*

ABOVE **Spinal problems can affect the whole body.**

RIGHT **A healthy spine allows free movement.**

Chiropractic is based on the belief that when bones become misaligned, muscles are thrown into spasm, causing immobility of ligaments and tendons, which in turn prevents the body from functioning properly. As a result, most body systems become impaired, and ill-health and pain result.

The body's healthy state is restored by moving the bones and joints back to their correct position. Chiropractors use force in order to move the joints and bones into place, but they do so with swift, practiced movements. All problems may have their root in structural imbalances. The spine is connected to the nervous system, which feeds every part of the body. Where there is pressure or

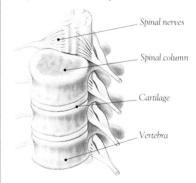

Spinal nerves

Spinal column

Cartilage

Vertebra

ABOVE **The spinal cord, containing the spinal nerves, connects with the brain.**

structural problems involving the spine, many different parts of the body may be affected, which can be manifested in illnesses as diverse as asthma, menstrual problems, headaches, sciatica, and behavioral problems.

Hippocrates (c.460–370 B.C.E.), the father of medicine, believed that knowledge of the spine was a prerequisite for understanding and treating numerous diseases. In later years, "bone-setters," or early chiropractors, were often successful in treating patients who could not be cured by the medical system of the time.

Where manipulation is involved, the chiropractor will use the correct amount of force at the correct speed to thrust into the spinal joint to the correct depth. There are more than 150 different chiropractic techniques commonly used.

HIPPOCRATES

TREATMENT

❋ Problems treated

All back and neck problems, including those caused by tension, injury, and congestion. Menstrual problems, headaches, asthma, pregnancy and post-natal problems, digestive and circulatory disorders, some heart conditions, insomnia, and constipation may also be resolved.

❋ Number of sessions necessary

You may need two or three sessions in the first few weeks, although occasionally one is all that is necessary. Treatment will last until the condition clears up, usually once or twice a month. You may come back for a "top-up" treatment twice a year after that.

BELOW **A chiropractor restores the spine to a perfectly functioning state.**

IS IT SAFE?

Chiropractic is safe for most people, although it is not recommended for some types of injury, and for people with conditions such as osteoporosis.

Specific movements are applied

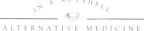
Healing

HEALING, *also called "spiritual healing," has, over the last few years, finally lost its mystical, magical associations. It has become one of the most important and popular means of alternative treatments available today.*

ABOVE **We may all have the power to heal.**

The scientific theory behind healing is still confused, and there are two main schools of thought. Some healers believe that a patient's brain waves are stimulated during the "healing" and that it is these waves that cause the healing process to take place, smoothing out imbalances within the body which might cause disease. Most healers, however, believe that they have been given a power that allows them to speed up the body's natural process of healing.

BELOW **Healing energy is believed to flow from the healer to the patient.**

We know that a wound heals naturally, or that the body eventually fights off infections. What healers do is accelerate this process in the body, with their powers. There is no question that spiritual healing works for many people – of all ages, and of all levels of health.

Our natural energies do become unbalanced by stress, poor diet, and negativity. Numerous adverse factors can block the healing mechanism so that it cannot function correctly, and we get ill. Spiritual healing provides the energy required to balance the body, mind, and spirit, and unblock the healing mechanism. A healer is effectively a channel for healing energy, which goes to the parts of the body where it is needed. Many healers believe that we all have the power to heal, if we choose to develop it.

Healing does not always work at a physical level: the illness may remain but the patient finds that his or her ability to cope with it improves. The healer effectively treats the whole person, removing an energy blockage, and promoting a feeling of relaxation.

The healer lays his or her hands on the body – sometimes in the air above it and occasionally on the affected area. Many patients report feeling a profound sensation – either hot or cold – which is replaced by a feeling of calm and well-being.

IS IT SAFE?

Healing is completely safe for people of any age or state of health.

TREATMENT

❋ **Problems treated**
Healing is used for many conditions, in particular stress and its associated symptoms. It is excellent for emotional disorders, musculo-skeletal disorders, serious medical conditions, and chronic illnesses. Some people have reported complete cures from terminal illnesses. Healing can be quite dramatic, when it works.

❋ **Number of sessions necessary**
Many healers require only one session, but the average number of sessions is between four and six.

Feeling of well-being

Healing energy is released

RIGHT **Patients usually feel very relaxed after a healing session.**

37

Homeopathy

HOMEOPATHY *is a complete system of medicine based on the theory that like is cured by like, which means that a substance that can produce symptoms of disease in a healthy person can cure the same symptoms in a sick person . It stimulates the body's defenses. Developed by the German physician Samuel Hahnemann (1755–1843), homeopathy is a holistic form of medicine that aims to help the body heal itself. It works for both acute (short-term) illnesses and chronic (long-term) ailments, and is concerned as much with preventing illness as it is with treatment.*

ABOVE **Belladonna** is often prescribed for sudden fevers.

Homeopathy is the opposite of conventional medicine. Instead of treating hay fever with drugs to suppress symptoms, a homeopath would treat it by introducing minute quantities of allergens which would encourage the body's immune response and allow it to heal itself. The minute substances used in treatment are called homeopathic remedies.

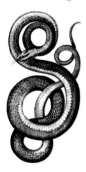

LEFT **The remedy Lachesis comes from snake venom.**

HOMEOPATHIC REMEDIES

Homeopathy uses preparations containing infinitesimal amounts of the original substance, diluted with milk, sugar, or alcohol, and succussed, or shaken. Remedies come in different potencies. To make a 6 potency, the substance is added to the diluter and succussed; the process is then repeated six times. A 30 potency has gone through the same

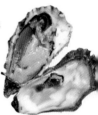

ABOVE **There are over 2,500 homeopathic remedies.**

HOMEOPATHIC DILUTION

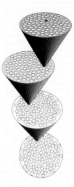

Remedies are made in different dilutions.

With each dilution, the remedy becomes more powerful.

The number on the remedy's label tells you how many dilutions have been made.

process 30 times. Although a 30 potency has been diluted more than a 6 potency, the succussion has made it more powerful and it is usually taken for more serious problems than a 6 potency.

Homeopathic remedies are prescribed for the whole person. A homeopath will consider your personal life, habits, emotions, diet, exercise, sleeping patterns, complexion, appetite, moods, libido, posture, environment, even the weather. The symptoms

themselves are analyzed carefully: their character is as important as the symptoms themselves and the constitution of the person experiencing them. Three people suffering muscle pain are likely to require three different remedies.

IS IT SAFE?

Homeopathic treatment is safe for people of all ages, including babies and children. However, only take remedies for as long as you need them.

TREATMENT

❋ **Problems treated**

Homeopathy can conceivably treat any condition, because it addresses every body system. It can be used in some emergency situations, such as shock or injury, when it offers remedies to encourage healing and to address the problem while you wait for conventional medical help. It tackles emotional conditions such as panic, anxiety, and fear, and most physical conditions.

❋ **Number of sessions necessary**

After your original consultation, you may need to return once or twice a month for your practitioner to assess the treatment, which may be adjusted as your symptoms change. Chronic conditions may require treatment over a long period of time; acute disorders may respond after one visit.

Hypnotherapy

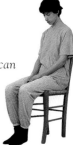

THE BRITISH MEDICAL ASSOCIATION *and the American Medical Association have tentatively defined hypnosis in part as "a temporary condition of altered attention in the subject that may be induced by another person." Although the condition resembles normal sleep, scientists have found that the brain-wave patterns of hypnotized subjects are much closer to the patterns of deep relaxation. Rather than being a psychic or mystical phenomenon, hypnosis is now generally viewed as a form of attentive, receptive, highly focused concentration in which external or peripheral events are omitted or disregarded.*

ABOVE **Under hypnotherapy, the brain shuts out external events.**

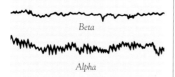

Beta

Alpha

ABOVE **Brain-wave patterns reveal the difference between ordinary and hypnotized states.**

Hypnotherapy involves making "suggestions" to a patient in a state of hypnosis. Subjects become quite unresponsive to ordinary forms of stimulation, and although they are told to sleep, they are also told to listen and to be ready to respond to commands or suggestions made by the hypnotist. Hypnosis is a tool for reaching and dealing with problems of the mind and body. In the hypnotized state, emotional problems can be addressed and resolved, and body functions can be improved to restore normal activity. There is evidence that hormonal problems, respiration, heart rate, circulation, and digestive activity can be influenced by hypnosis, and many people find they can cut off completely from sensations of pain.

Hypnotherapists believe that the mind has the power to create any disease known to man – and the power to cure it by activating the healing and repair mechanism, which is controlled by the subconscious mind.

Hypnotherapists reach the subconscious by inducing a trance in the subject, which can be light, medium, or deep.

LEFT *The mind is the key to the health of the body.*

Therapists begin the process by encouraging you to relax. There are several way of doing this: the most common is through the use of your imagination.

Hypnohealing is aimed at healing pathological disease. The therapist helps you uncover the cause of your illness and, through visualization, encourages you to release it.

Cell command therapy, or "cellular regeneration," is a similar technique, used to slow down ageing and associated degenerative diseases.

IS IT SAFE?

Regardless of the application, hypnosis should be left to those who are properly trained. When used by untrained persons, it may have undesirable and even dangerous effects.

TREATMENT

❋ Problems treated

Hypnotherapy is especially useful in the treatment of behavioral and habitual difficulties, such as smoking, eating disorders, phobias, etc. Other conditions treated include arthritis, asthma, digestive troubles, eczema, insomnia, migraine, stress, and many childhood problems such as colic, bed-wetting, and hyperactivity. It is very good for chronic pain, such as sciatica and headaches. Some cancers respond to treatment.

❋ Number of sessions necessary

This depends on the length of time you have had your condition and its seriousness. In general, some treatments are effective after one or two sessions; others require up to 15 or 20 sessions for full healing.

RIGHT *Hypnotherapy begins with complete relaxation.*

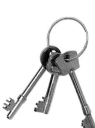

Naturopathy

ORGANIC FOOD

NATUROPATHY IS, *like Ayurveda, more than just a therapy: it is a philosophy for living. It is based on the belief that the body has the ability to heal itself when free of the toxins that are accumulated through poor lifestyle habits. Naturopathy stimulates the body's natural defenses and promotes an equilibrium that allows it to function properly and effectively.*

PHILOSOPHY

Naturopaths believe that four basic components make for good health:

- Clean air.
- Clean water.
- Clean food from good earth.
- Exercise and healthy living.

Naturopathic treatments work with the above elements to restore health and well-being. Naturopaths believe that getting ill is natural, and that methods of cure should follow the same natural principles. Symptoms of illness are encouraged to come out, while the body resists and finds its proper balance. Naturopaths also routinely encourage brief fasting to get over simple infections such as flu, and will pay a great deal of attention to bowel health.

Naturopaths usually follow three main principles:

1 The body has the power to heal itself, so treatment should not be given to alleviate symptoms, but to support the healing power of nature.

2 The symptoms of disease are not part of the disease itself but a sign that the body is striving to eliminate toxins and return to its natural state of balance.

3 All treatments should be holistic.

RIGHT **Regain your vitality.**

Naturopathic treatments include:

- Breathing – long, deep breaths to expand the ribcage; the use of ionizers.
- Hydrotherapy – the use of water to promote healing, improve circulation, stimulate energy, ease pain, reduce fever, soothe the nervous system, and empty the bowels.
- Baths – including Turkish baths, spa baths, saunas.
- Douches – hot and cold water sprays on specific areas of the body.
- Compresses – hot and cold.
- Enemas – the internal use of water to cleanse the lower bowel.

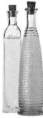

BATH OILS

- Colonic irrigation – flushing out toxic waste and impacted feces from further up the bowel, in the colon.
- Diet – eating foods that have not been processed or refined, and which are mostly organic. Naturopaths believe such foods fuel vitality and stimulate the vital force.
- Fasting – in order to cleanse

TREATMENT

❋ **Problems treated**
Naturopathy can help with a wide range of acute and chronic problems, such as anemia, allergies, arthritis, circulation disorders, constipation, cystitis, eczema and other skin diseases, hangovers, irritable bowel syndrome, migraine, pre-menstrual syndrome, ulcers, and varicose veins.

❋ **Number of sessions necessary**
Treatment may go on for some time, depending on the severity of your condition and the length of time you have had it. Naturopaths aim to educate you so that new, good habits will prevent future illness and improve vitality. Some patients see their practitioner regularly, long after the original complaint has been resolved.

IS IT SAFE?

Because naturopathy is multidisciplined, there is a therapy or a course of treatment for everyone, and each program will be tailor-made for the individual. Ensure that your therapist is trained and qualified.

the system of poisons accumulated from bad eating habits, a poor environment, and suppressed or repressed emotions; to enhance immune functioning and speed up healing, and to give the digestive system a rest.

- Osteopathy, homeopathy, and a range of other treatments.

Nutritional therapy

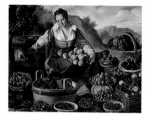

ABOVE **Nature's harvest – in a pre-pesticide age.**

NUTRITIONAL THERAPY *is the use of food and the diet to treat and prevent illness, and to restore the body to its natural, healthy equilibrium. Food has always been used for its medicinal effects, and we now know that a varied diet, rich in natural ingredients, is essential for good health. Diet is an integral element in almost all therapies.*

In today's world, intensive farming methods, pollution, pesticides, and refining processes make our diets often far less nutritious than they appear. Alcohol, tobacco, drugs, and stress also rob the body of nutrients. Nutritional therapy is based on the belief that the body is made up of elements that were once the nutritional elements of food. The idea is that health problems crop up when one of the nutritional links is weak or missing. The nutritional therapist decides how it can be put back in place, using nutrition and supplements.

Possible food allergies or intolerance may be identified,

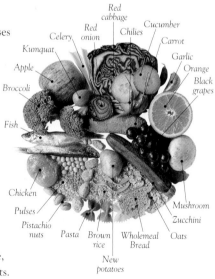

Red cabbage
Celery
Red onion
Chilies
Cucumber
Carrot
Kumquat
Garlic
Apple
Orange
Black grapes
Broccoli
Fish
Chicken
Pulses
Mushroom
Zucchini
Pistachio nuts
Pasta
Brown rice
Wholemeal Bread
Oats
New potatoes

ABOVE **A varied, balanced diet is an important weapon against disease.**

and extra foods suggested to provide therapeutic benefits. Treatment will always be strictly tailored to the individual.

Elements of nutrition that can be used as health supplements include: vitamins, minerals, amino acids, nucleic acids and derivatives, lipids and derivatives, herbs, acidophilus, bioflavonoids, yeast, co-enzyme Q10, enzymes, glandulars, hyaluronic acid, oxygen therapies, testosterone and steroids, fruit acids, charcoal, bee and flower pollen, royal jelly, seaweeds and derivatives, spirulina chlorella, lipoic acid.

IS IT SAFE?

Supplementation should always be supervised by a qualified therapist, because megadosing on one can upset the fine balance in the body. Some supplements are toxic in excess. There are special treatments designed for pregnant women, children, babies, the elderly, and people with long-term, chronic conditions.

TREATMENT

✤ Problems treated

Most conditions, such as anxiety, arthritis, asthma, depression, digestive disorders, eczema, headaches, herpes, high blood-pressure, hormone problems, PMS, osteoporosis, pregnancy problems, reduced immunities, skin problems, stress, and viruses. Most importantly, nutritional therapy is preventive.

✤ Number of sessions necessary

This will be dependent on the severity of the condition and the length of time you have had it. You'll notice the benefits as soon as dietary changes are made, but long-term illness may take up to 10 sessions to clear.

✤ Long-term effects

All systems of your body will be improved to the point of optimum heath, and in a fit state you are more likely to fight off infection and deal efficiently with any health problems or injury.

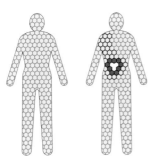

LEFT *Elements of nutrition combine to form a barrier against ill-health.*

Osteopathy

OSTEOPATHY *is a therapy based on manipulation of bones and muscles. Osteopaths maintain that the normal, healthy body produces forces necessary to fight disease, and that most ailments are due to the misalignment of bones and other faulty conditions of the muscle tissue and cartilage.*

A PERFECT SPECIMEN?

Osteopathy was developed in the U.S. in 1874 by Andrew Taylor Still, as a reaction to the primitive conditions and surgical techniques he had observed during the American Civil War. He fully believed that medical treatment should be holistic (treating the whole person, not just the affected parts). This theory still underlies the discipline today.

Osteopathic medicine is based on the belief that the body will manufacture its own remedies and defenses against disease, if the musculoskeletal structure is in correct mechanical adjustment. When the spine and skeleton are misaligned, organs may not function properly, and blood and lymphatic fluid circulation is impaired. By restoring balance and correcting any lesions or misalignment, blood can flow

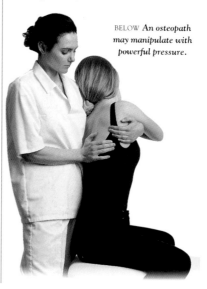

BELOW **An osteopath may manipulate with powerful pressure.**

smoothly to the organs, the nervous system is able to function properly, and the lymphatic system is free of any stagnation that can cause toxins to build up. Digestion, respiration, and every other body process will be improved as a result of treatment.

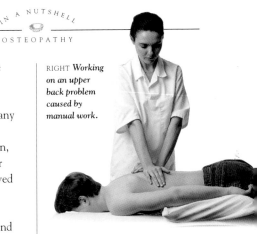

RIGHT *Working on an upper back problem caused by manual work.*

Treatment consists of stretching, manipulation, and often quite powerful pressure, to relax the soft tissues and muscles of the body. Joints are exercised to improve flexibility, and pressure is applied to areas where there is misalignment.

Cranio-sacral technique involves gently massaging the bones and muscles of the cranium (skull) and the sacrum (base of the spine) in order to improve the flow of cerebro-spinal fluid, which bathes the nervous system. The release of tension created by this technique will affect functions throughout the body.

IS IT SAFE?

Osteopathy can be safe for people of any age or level of health, but some conditions, including inflammatory diseases or bone conditions such as osteoporosis, contraindicate its use.

TREATMENT

❋ **Problems treated**
Back and neck troubles, musculo-skeletal pain, circulation, breathing problems, depression, digestive disorders, constipation, migraine, fatigue, inflammation, joint pain, nausea, neuralgia, sciatica, some skin problems, menstrual and pre-menstrual disorders, stress, and eczema. Energy levels and well-being will be restored to optimum levels.

❋ **Number of sessions necessary**
Three to five sessions are usually enough to correct the majority of problems, although long-term or chronic illnesses may require more treatments. Some patients like to return for follow-up treatment to benefit from the realignment.

Reflexology

REFLEXOLOGY *involves stimulating, massaging, and applying pressure to points on the hands and feet that correspond to various systems and organs throughout the body, to stimulate the body's own healing system. These points are called "reflex points," and each point corresponds to a different body part or function.*

Reflexologists believe that applying pressure to reflex points will stimulate the body to heal itself.

Pressure applied to nerve endings can influence all the body systems, including the circulation and lymphatic systems. Improvements here result in improved body functioning, because nutrients

RIGHT **Reflexology can ease tension and reduce inflammation.**

and oxygen are transported more efficiently round the body and toxins are eliminated with greater ease.

Reflexologists believe that the body is divided into ten vertical zones or channels, five

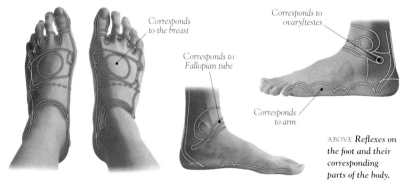

Corresponds to the breast

Corresponds to Fallopian tube

Corresponds to ovary/testes

Corresponds to arm

ABOVE **Reflexes on the foot and their corresponding parts of the body.**

on the left and five on the right. Each zone runs from the head right down to the reflex areas on the hands and feet, and from the front through to the back of the body. All the body parts within any one zone are linked by the nerve pathways and are mirrored in the corresponding reflex zone on the hands and feet. By applying pressure to a reflex point or area, the therapist can stimulate or rebalance the energy in the related zone.

Each zone is a channel for energy (called chi in Eastern disciplines). For example, working a zone on the foot, linked with the kidneys, will release vital energy that may be blocked somewhere else in that zone, such as in the eyes. Working the kidney reflex area on the foot will therefore revitalize and balance the entire zone and improve functioning of the organ.

RIGHT **Pressure applied to a reflex point stimulates the related zone.**

IS IT SAFE?

Reflexology is safe for everyone, although some conditions, such as pregnancy, may call for different treatment, and some reflex points will need to be avoided.

TREATMENT

❈ **Problems treated**
Reflexology is an excellent whole-body system, and can be used both to prevent illness and to encourage the body to heal. It is particularly useful for stress and related disorders, emotional disorders, digestive problems, circulatory disorders, menstrual problems, insomnia, fatigue, and most chronic and acute illnesses.

❈ **Number of sessions necessary**
Treatment varies according to the problem and the length of time you have had it; some people require treatment two or three times in quick succession, slowing down to once a month or even less often. Many people continue to have treatment after the original problem is resolved, in order to keep the body balanced.

Releases energy

Pressure from thumbs

Western herbalism

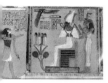

ABOVE **The Ancient Egyptians had many herbal remedies.**

HERBALISM *is probably the oldest recorded form of medicine, beginning in ancient cultures more than 5,000 years ago. Western herbalism combines the ancient teachings of the East with indigenous traditions and folk remedies, complemented by modern-day scientific study.*

The term "herb" includes any plant, and any part of a plant, that can be used to make a remedy. This can include seaweeds, ferns, flowers, roots, bulbs, barks, seeds, and leaves. It includes cooking herbs, spices, and many fruits and vegetables.

ARCTIUM LAPPA

Herbalism is the use of plants as medicines to restore and maintain health by keeping the body in balance. It relies on specific qualities of individual plants to stimulate the body's healing system and restore health. Like most holistic practitioners, herbalists believe that we all possess healing energy, which they call the "vital force." This vital force works constantly to maintain our holistic health – that is, health on spiritual, physical, and emotional levels. When our vital force is weakened by stress,

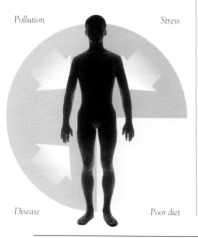

Pollution

Stress

Disease

Poor diet

LEFT **Our vital force, or healing energy, is constantly under attack.**

disease, poor diet, or pollution, we begin to show signs of disease. Symptoms – which conventional medicine tends to suppress with drugs – are, to a herbalist, an indication that the body is trying to fight the illness on its own.

QUALITIES OF HERBS

Herbs can have many properties. They are antibacterial, antiviral, anti-fungal, sedative, relaxing, tonic, nervine, carminative, restorative, stimulant, insecticidal, among others.

Herbal remedies are prescribed to support the affected body systems in their fight against disease. The purpose of the herbs, therefore, is not only to alleviate disease, but also to prevent it recurring; to detoxify the system of poisons that can cause disease; and to support the immune system and maintain balance.

In any form, herbs are prescribed for an individual to address the cause of a health problem, and any imbalances within the body. In this way, future illnesses will be prevented, the immune system will be

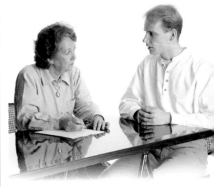

ABOVE *Give your herbalist as complete a picture as possible.*

stimulated, and symptoms will be eased as the condition is resolved by the body. There are thousands of herbs available, with extensive properties, and it is highly recommended that you seek advice, diagnosis, and treatment from a registered practitioner.

LEFT *Iris rhizome is used to treat inflammation.*

IRIS

There are several major ways of preparing herbs:

• **Infusions** are prepared by steeping fresh or dried herbs in boiling water and employing the liquid for external or internal use.

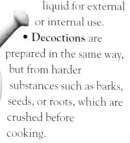

PESTLE AND MORTAR

• **Decoctions** are prepared in the same way, but from harder substances such as barks, seeds, or roots, which are crushed before cooking.

• **Powders** may be prepared from crushed herbs, barks, seeds, and stems.

• **Capsules and tablets** are made from powders.

CAPSULES

• **Syrup** is made from a decoction or an infusion, which is boiled with honey and other herbal syrup to create a herbal preparation.

BAI JIAO HUI XIANG

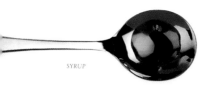

SYRUP

• **Tinctures** are herbs suspended in alcohol, into which the active properties of the herbs are released.

MASSAGE OIL

• **Essential oils** (see aromatherapy) are usually extracted by distillation or compression. They may also be used for massage.

• **Suppositories** are sometimes prescribed for rectal problems such as piles.

• **Douches** may be prescribed for vaginal infections.

• **Herbal baths** are an excellent herbal treatment and involve tying a handful of herbs in a muslin bag, and hanging it from the bath faucet so that the water runs through it.

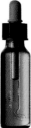

ESSENTIAL OIL

• **Ointments, creams, compresses, and poultices** can be applied directly to affected areas to allow the active ingredients of the plant to work.

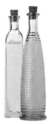

BATH TREATMENT

The skill of a herbalist lies in his or her ability to choose exactly the right herb combination – suited to your specific constitution and symptoms. Many health professionals run seminars or work in health stores, and they will be able to advise you which remedy might be appropriate for you, if you aren't sure which one to use.

BELOW *Herbal tea, such as peppermint, makes a refreshing change. It is naturally caffeine-free.*

ROSE PETALS

TREATMENT

❉ Problems treated

Herbal medicine treats the same range of conditions that conventional medicine treats. However, in medical emergencies, such as serious injury, acute illness involving the organs or skeleton, or in cases of serious infection or disease, you must always seek urgent conventional medical attention. Herbalism is particularly good for longer-term, chronic conditions such as allergies, asthma, cystitis, depression, digestive disorders, neuralgia, menstrual problems, respiratory problems, skin problems, stress, and viral infections.

❉ Number of sessions necessary

Acute (short-term) illnesses may respond quickly, and be resolved in two or three sessions. Chronic or long-term conditions may take several weeks or months for a cure to be effected. Sessions may take place about once a week to begin with, reducing to once or twice every few months thereafter.

IS IT SAFE?

Herbs can be toxic in large quantities, and many herbs are contraindicated in pregnancy, for children, and in some medical conditions. All remedies must be prudently administered, and your therapist must be aware of any other treatments you are receiving.

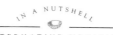
Self-help for common ailments

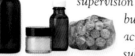

MANY ALTERNATIVE *therapies can be undertaken at home, although it is usually suggested that you do so only under the supervision of an experienced practitioner. It is easy to buy remedies from your local health store, or across the counter at the pharmacy, but their subtle variations can only be discerned by a professional. For example, there are probably over two dozen herbs that could be used to treat indigestion.*

Some types of remedy, such as aromatherapy oils, pre-packaged herbs, and homeopathic remedies are available in shops, and you can choose and administer them yourself. Always read the label before taking any medication.

The following pages outline the therapies that are suitable for the complaints listed. The success of a treatment will be dependent upon the individual condition.

HOW TO USE THESE CHARTS

Read across to select appropriate therapies.

Health problem

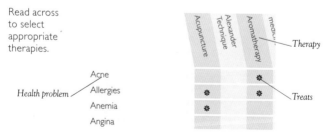

	Acupuncture	Alexander Technique	Aromatherapy	*medic...*
Acne			✹	*Therapy*
Allergies	✹		✹	*Treats*
Anemia	✹			
Angina				

	Acne	Allergies	Anemia	Angina	Arteriosclerosis	Arthritis and rheumatism	Asthma	Backache	Bad breath (halitosis)	Breaks and fractures	Cataracts	Catarrh	Cellulite	Chilblains	Chronic bronchitis	Cold sores	Colds	Conjunctivitis
Western herbalism	✽	✽	✽		✽	✽	✽		✽	✽		✽	✽	✽	✽	✽	✽	✽
Reflexology				✽	✽	✽	✽					✽			✽		✽	
Osteopathy						✽		✽					✽		✽			
Nutritional therapy	✽	✽	✽	✽	✽	✽	✽		✽		✽	✽	✽	✽		✽	✽	✽
Naturopathy	✽	✽		✽	✽	✽			✽			✽	✽	✽	✽	✽	✽	✽
Hypnotherapy	✽	✽					✽											
Homeopathy	✽	✽	✽	✽		✽	✽		✽	✽	✽		✽			✽	✽	✽
Healing			✽						✽	✽								
Chiropractic						✽		✽										
Chinese herbalism	✽	✽	✽	✽	✽		✽		✽			✽			✽	✽	✽	✽
Bach Flower Remedies	✽							✽										
Ayurvedic medicine		✽			✽	✽	✽	✽				✽			✽	✽		✽
Aromatherapy	✽	✽				✽		✽	✽			✽	✽	✽	✽	✽	✽	
Alexander Technique						✽		✽										
Acupuncture		✽	✽			✽	✽	✽	✽	✽					✽	✽		✽	✽

	Constipation	Coughs	Cramp	Cystitis	Dandruff	Depression	Diabetes	Diarrhea	Ear infections	Eczema	Gallstones	Glandular fever	Hair loss and baldness	Hangover	Hay fever	Headaches	Hemorrhoids	Hodgkin's Disease
Western herbalism	✽	✽		✽	✽	✽		✽	✽	✽	✽	✽		✽	✽	✽	✽	
Reflexology	✽			✽		✽			✽	✽	✽	✽	✽	✽		✽	✽	✽
Osteopathy	✽			✽			✽		✽						✽	✽		
Nutritional therapy	✽		✽	✽	✽		✽	✽		✽		✽	✽	✽		✽		✽
Naturopathy	✽			✽		✽	✽		✽	✽	✽	✽		✽		✽		
Hypnotherapy	✽			✽		✽		✽		✽			✽			✽	✽	
Homeopathy	✽	✽	✽	✽	✽	✽	✽	✽	✽	✽	✽	✽	✽		✽	✽	✽	✽
Healing		✽		✽		✽			✽				✽					✽
Chiropractic			✽	✽		✽				✽						✽		
Chinese herbalism	✽	✽		✽		✽	✽	✽	✽	✽		✽	✽	✽	✽	✽	✽	
Bach Flower Remedies						✽				✽						✽		
Ayurvedic medicine	✽	✽		✽	✽		✽		✽			✽	✽		✽		✽	✽
Aromatherapy		✽	✽	✽		✽		✽	✽	✽	✽				✽			
Alexander Technique						✽						✽			✽	✽		
Acupuncture	✽	✽				✽	✽	✽	✽	✽	✽	✽		✽	✽	✽	✽	

	Hyperactivity	I.B.S.	Impetigo	Indigestion	Influenza	Insomnia	Kidney stones	M.E.	Menopause symptoms	Nausea and vomiting	Neuralgia	Obesity	Osteoporosis	P.M.S. and period problems	Pneumonia	Psoriasis	Raynaud's Phenomenon	Shingles
Western herbalism		❋	❋	❋	❋	❋	❋	❋		❋		❋	❋	❋	❋	❋	❋	❋
Reflexology		❋	❋	❋	❋	❋		❋		❋		❋		❋		❋	❋	
Osteopathy	❋			❋										❋				
Nutritional therapy	❋	❋	❋		❋	❋	❋	❋	❋	❋			❋	❋		❋	❋	❋
Naturopathy	❋	❋	❋	❋	❋	❋	❋		❋		❋		❋	❋	❋			❋
Hypnotherapy			❋			❋	❋	❋		❋	❋	❋	❋	❋				
Homeopathy	❋	❋	❋	❋	❋	❋	❋	❋	❋	❋	❋	❋	❋	❋	❋	❋	❋	❋
Healing			❋		❋							❋	❋	❋				
Chiropractic	❋			❋		❋			❋				❋	❋				
Chinese herbalism		❋		❋	❋	❋	❋	❋	❋				❋	❋	❋	❋	❋	❋
Bach Flower Remedies	❋	❋	❋	❋														
Ayurvedic medicine	❋		❋	❋	❋	❋			❋		❋		❋	❋	❋	❋	❋	❋
Aromatherapy		❋	❋			❋	❋		❋		❋		❋	❋			❋	❋
Alexander Technique	❋	❋		❋	❋			❋					❋					
Acupuncture	❋	❋		❋	❋				❋	❋			❋	❋		❋	❋	❋

	Sinus problems	Sprains	Stress	Thrush	Thyroid problems	Tonsillitis	Ulcers (peptic)	Urticaria	Varicose veins	Warts
Western herbalism	✽	✽	✽	✽	✽	✽	✽	✽	✽	✽
Reflexology	✽		✽		✽	✽	✽		✽	
Osteopathy		✽	✽							
Nutritional therapy	✽	✽	✽	✽	✽	✽		✽	✽	
Naturopathy	✽		✽	✽		✽	✽	✽	✽	
Hypnotherapy				✽			✽		✽	
Homeopathy	✽	✽	✽	✽	✽	✽	✽	✽	✽	✽
Healing		✽		✽						
Chiropractic	✽		✽			✽				
Chinese herbalism	✽		✽	✽	✽	✽	✽	✽		✽
Bach Flower Remedies		✽	✽				✽	✽		
Ayurvedic medicine	✽			✽	✽		✽	✽		
Aromatherapy	✽	✽	✽	✽		✽			✽	
Alexander Technique	✽		✽					✽		
Acupuncture		✽		✽			✽	✽		✽

Further reading

THE COMPLETE FAMILY GUIDE TO
ALTERNATIVE MEDICINE (Element
Books, 1996)

Inge Dougans, THE COMPLETE
ILLUSTRATED GUIDE TO REFLEXOLOGY
(Element Books, 1996)

Dr Christopher Hammond, THE
COMPLETE FAMILY GUIDE TO
HOMEOPATHY (Element Books, 1995)

David Hoffmann, THE COMPLETE
ILLUSTRATED HOLISTIC HERBAL
(Element Books, 1996)

Julia Lawless, THE COMPLETE
ILLUSTRATED ENCYCLOPEDIA OF
ESSENTIAL OILS (Element Books, 1995)

Tom Williams, THE COMPLETE
ILLUSTRATED GUIDE TO CHINESE
MEDICINE (Element Books, 1996)

Useful addresses

**British Complementary
Medicine Association**
39 Prestbury Road
Cheltenham
Glos GL52 2PT
United Kingdom

British Homeopathic Association
27A Devonshire Street
London W1N 1RJ
United Kingdom

**American Association of
Oriental Medicine**
433 Front Street
Catasauqua
Pennsylvania 18032
U.S.A.

**American Foundation
for Homeopathy**
1508 S Garfield
Alhambra CA 91801
U.S.A.

American Herbalists Guild
PO Box 1683
Soquel CA 95073
U.S.A.

**Australian Federation
of Homeopathy**
PO Box 806
Spit Junction NSW 2088
Australia

**Australian Natural
Therapists' Association Ltd**
PO Box 522
Sutherland NSW 2232
Australia

**Australian Traditional Medicine
Society Limited**
PO Box 1027 (mailing)
12/27 Bank Street (office)
Meadowbank NSW 2114
Australia